Move Happy

Healthy, playful movement adventures for humans

David McGuigan and Laura McGuigan

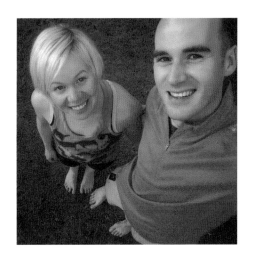

Laura does the pics. Dave does the words.

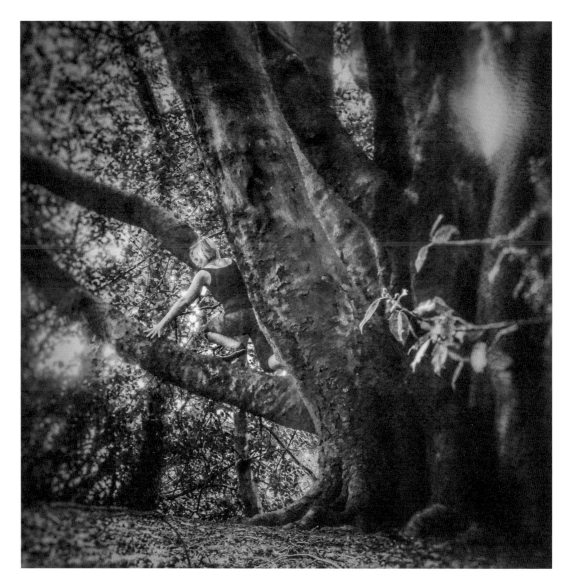

adventure
(noun)
an unusual, exciting or daring experience

move happy

When was the last time you had an adventure?

In the modern world of sports and gyms, it may seem unusual to wish to move as we were designed, in settings we were designed to move in. These are the old ways, surely of no use to us today. But perhaps we're becoming disconnected. What if moving more naturally is just the thing we need more of to help improve our health & wellbeing?

Our aim in Move Happy is to get you excited about natural human movement. To marvel at how playful and joyous it can be. To seek opportunities to move, to reconnect to your human nature and learn new things about yourself. Rediscovering your ability to move more naturally is an adventure in itself, one that we believe can last an entire lifetime.

We'll begin by sharing some of the basics with you and build slowly from there. As you make your way through the book you'll see that it's all free to try, the ability is largely already in you and you can go at a pace that suits you right the way through. Ultimately we aim to help you reach a point where you can fill each day with mini movement adventures of your own.

Your role will be to dare to get out there and make that first move. You might need to be brave; not just to see what you are capable of, but maybe to question some of the conventions you currently live by. Like putting yourself in situations where you could get bumped and a little dirty, perhaps even restoring some of that curiosity and playfulness you had as a child.

So, how would you like to come with us and start a new adventure today?

breathe

"Another glorious day, the air
as delicious to the lungs as
a nectar to the tongue."

— John Muir

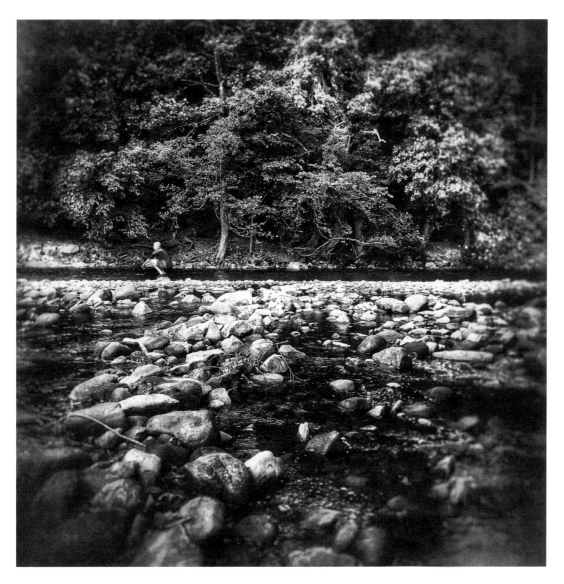

Before we start on our movement adventure, take a moment to find a quiet spot and just be still. Try to pay a little attention to your surroundings and yourself.
Feel yourself breathing.

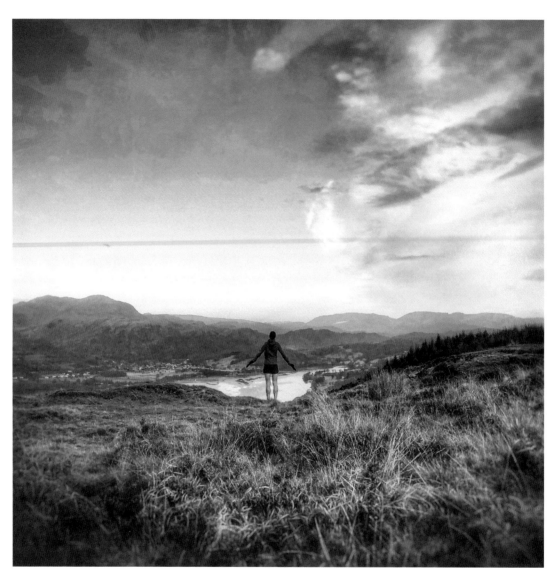

Breathing is the most primal and primary of all human functions. It happens whether you notice it or not. It is movement in its purest form. Try taking a nice deep breath in right now, letting your lungs fill with oxygen rich air.

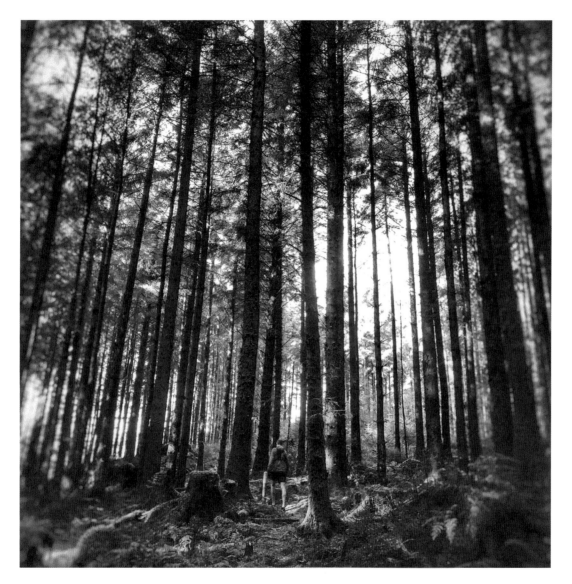

The oxygen is transferred to your blood, where it is transported to provide nourishment to every corner of your body. When you breathe out the cycle completes, ready to begin again. This movement is the continual process of life.

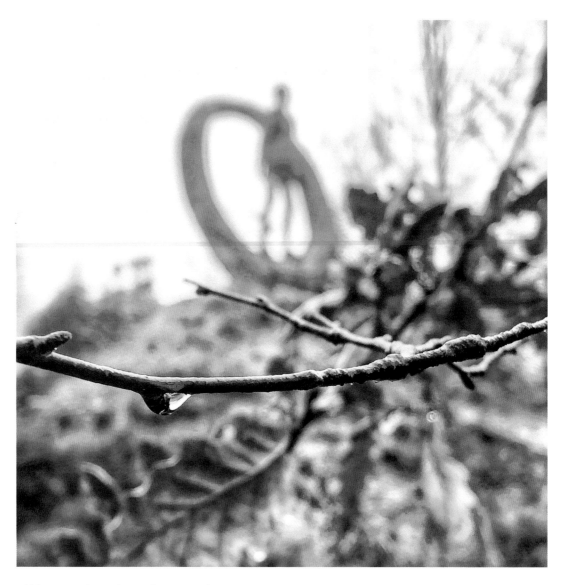

When you breathe well your entire torso expands and contracts with ease. You feel calm, poised and ready to act. Short, shallow breathing can make you feel anxious and agitated, like you're holding on to something - scared to act.

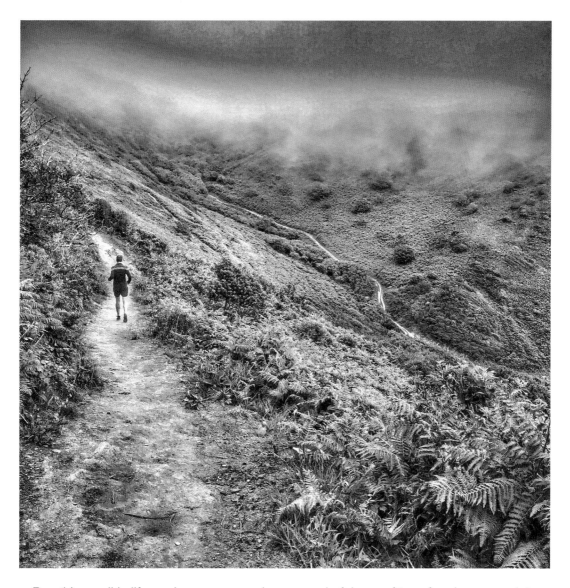

Breathing well in life, and as you move, has a wonderful way of transforming nerves into excitement. This movement adventure is meant to be exciting.
If you get stuck at any point, the first thing to remember is to breathe.

walk

"Let him who would move
the world first move himself."

— Socrates

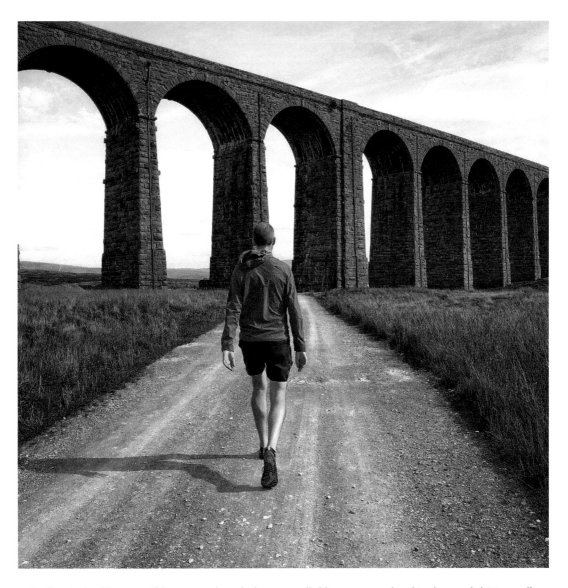

Let's start with something you already know well. Humans evolved to be upright to walk - it's wired into your DNA. Your biggest early life adventure was to pull yourself to your feet and walk. You were naturally curious and wanted to explore.

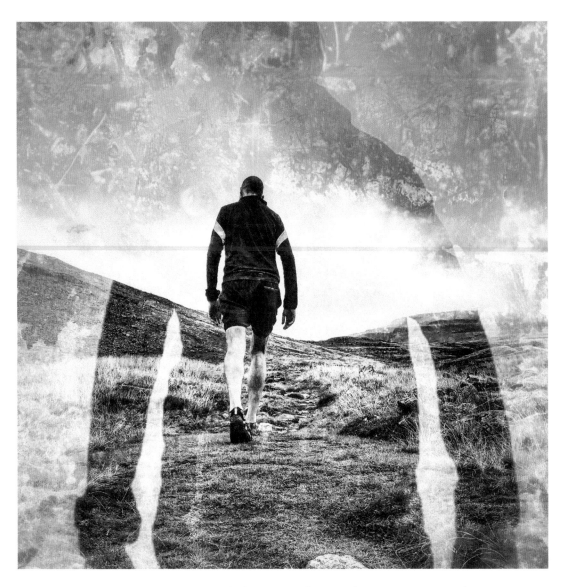

Walking in nature across varied terrain delivers a deep sensory experience.
Look around as you go. Take it all in. Listen, smell, touch, breathe.

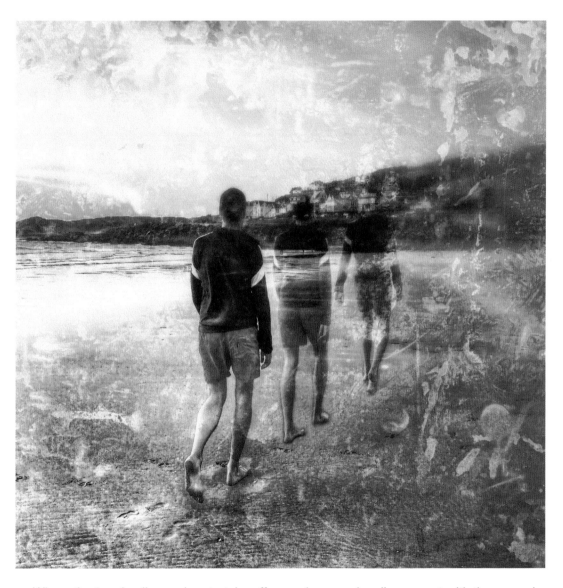

Where the terrain allows, dare to take off your shoes and really connect with the ground.
Feel the energy and support the Earth provides from head to toe.

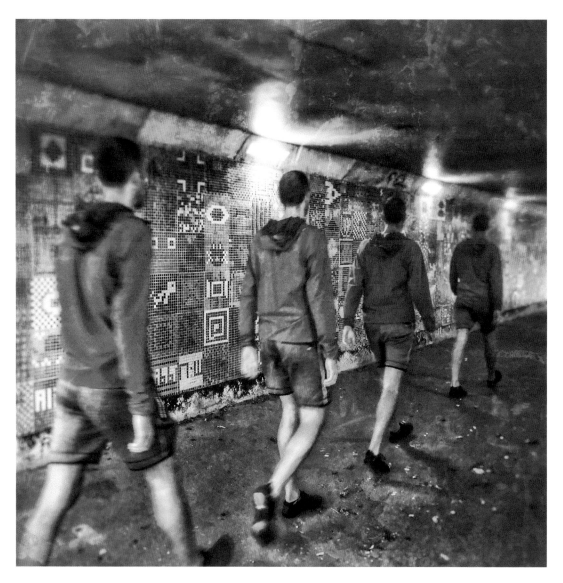

Creative places and problem solving spaces. Allow your mind to wander along with you as you walk. It's amazing where it will go if you let it.

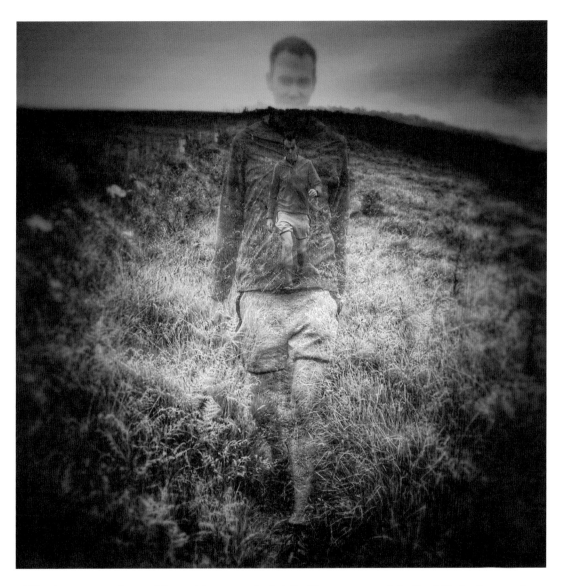

Whether you make walking a bigger part of daily life or escape into the hills for hours at a time, praise yourself for creating the space in your busy schedule to do it. Then make walking the reward.

hurdle

"If you can find a path
without obstacles, it probably
doesn't lead anywhere."

— Frank A Clark

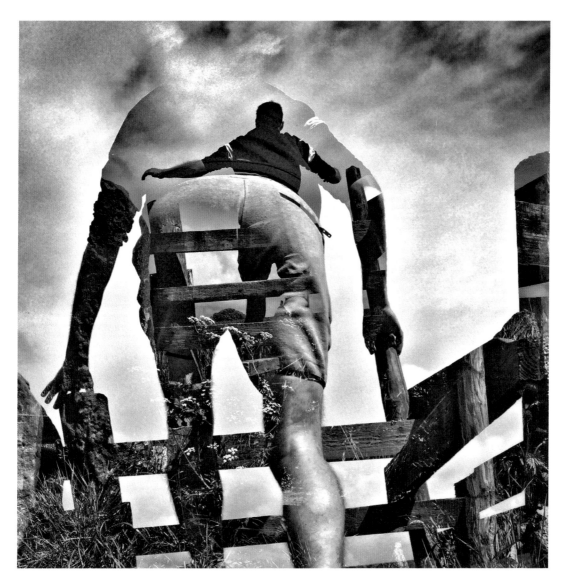

On your walks, as in life, there will be obstacles along the way.

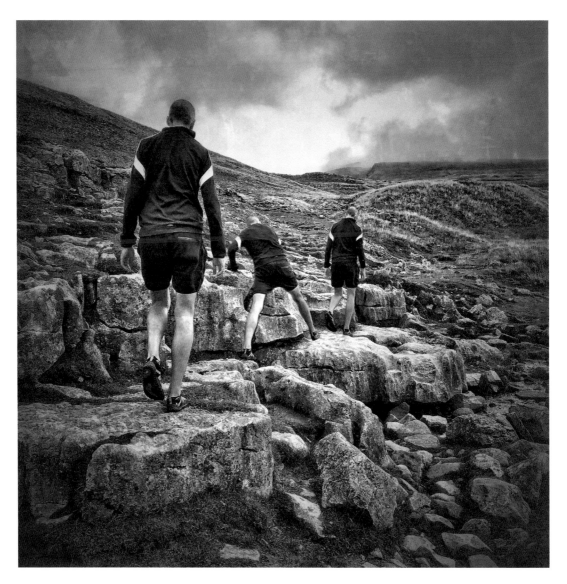

Some of these obstacles will be natural; like mountains, rivers or rocks.

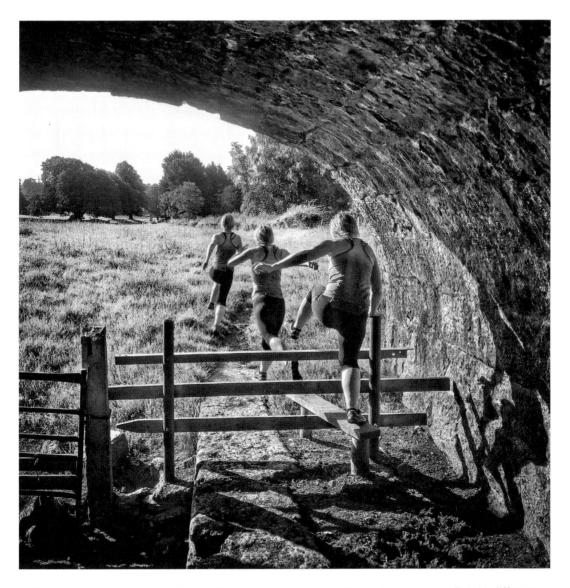

Some will be man made; like walls, gates and fences. They all represent slightly different challenges - opportunities to add new movements.

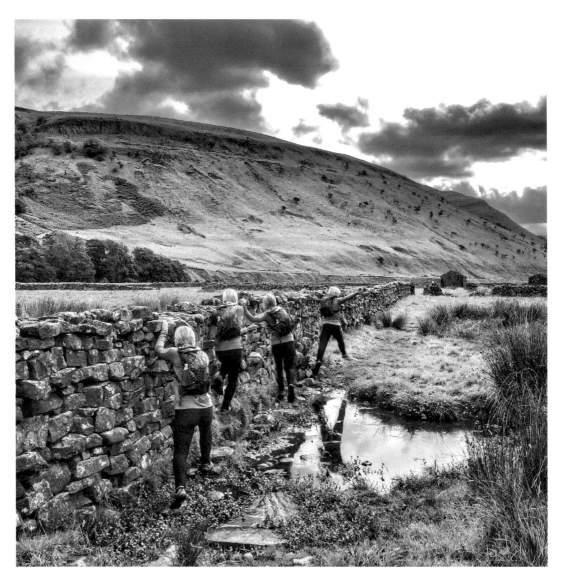

Use your body, mind and whatever else is around to help you to overcome them.

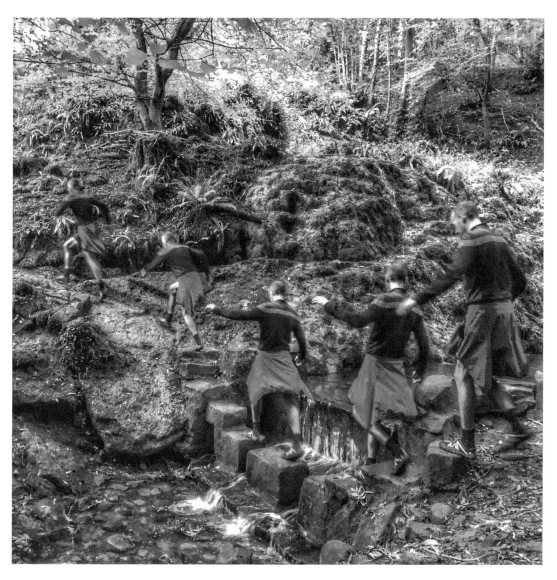

Allow yourself a small smile of contentment when you clear an obstacle and continue on your adventure without missing a step.

climb

"If growing up means it would
be beneath my dignity to
climb a tree, I'll never grow up."

— J.M Barrie

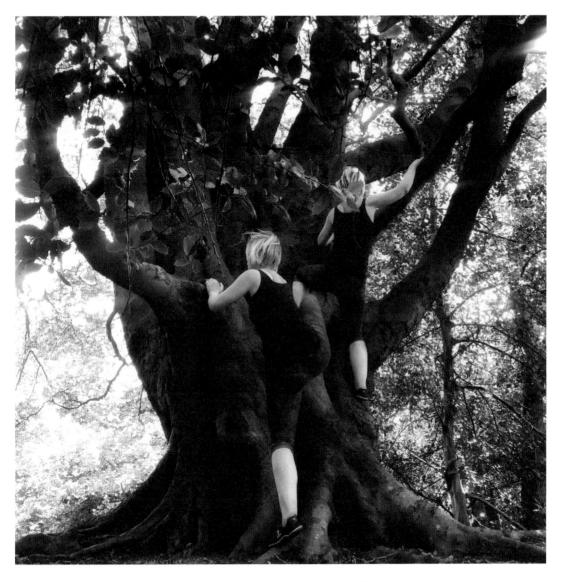

You're not aiming to become a world class climber here. It's not about how high you go or how technical the route, but about reaching up, making the first move and seeing where it takes you.

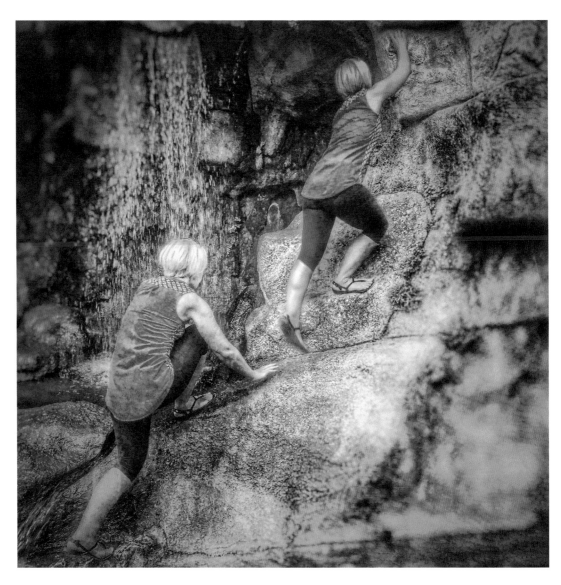

It's not about expensive technical equipment either. All you need is you.

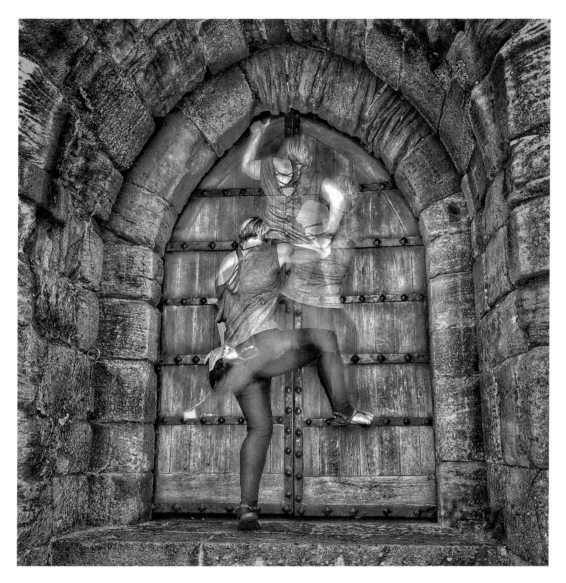

You and your ability to not only spot climbing opportunities, but take them too. Young children are masters of this game. They don't ask questions, they just go for it. Watch what they do and follow their lead.

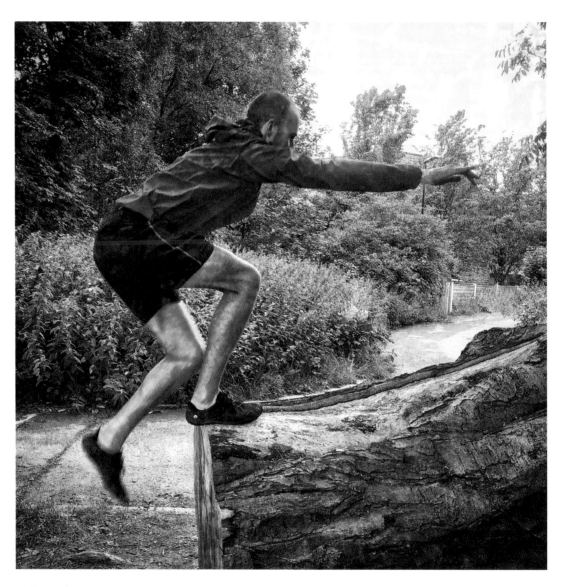

One of the reasons climbing is so great is because your whole body gets involved. Even when you think you aren't using your hands, you probably are.

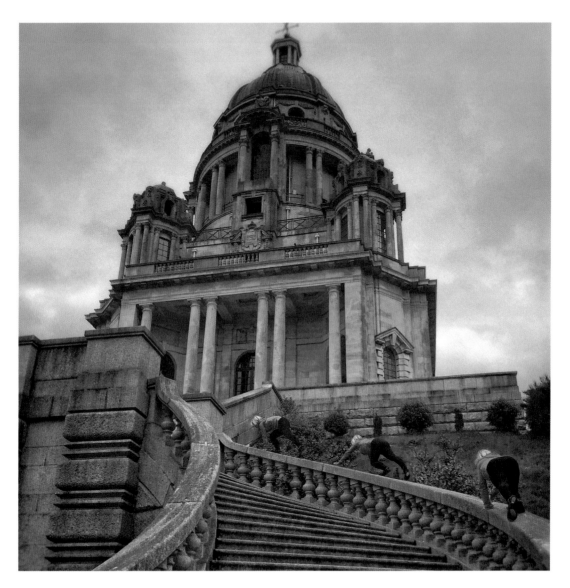

You're now beginning to step beyond some of the accepted norms of adult behaviour. It's easy to take the clearest route, but the real fun can often be found off the beaten track.

balance

"The greatest victory is that
which requires no battle."

— Sun Tzu

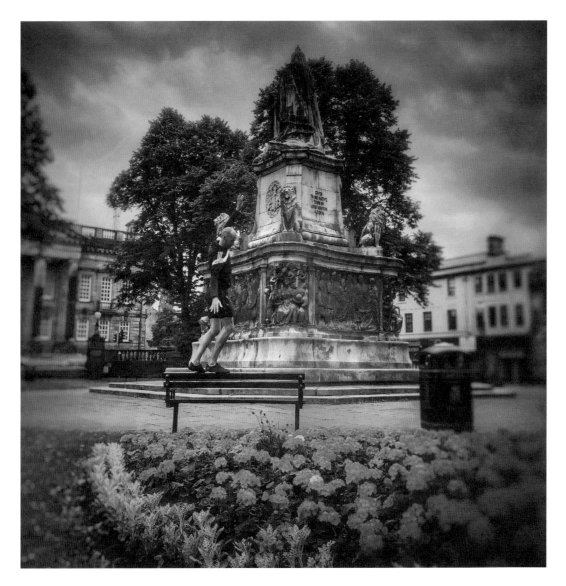

Balance is required in every form of human movement. Yet the perfectly engineered surfaces of the modern world mean you rarely get the chance to connect with and challenge your sense of balance.

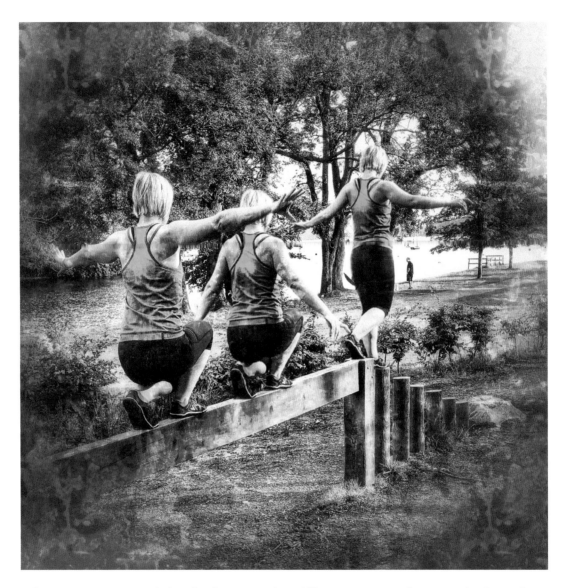

As you may suspect, balancing is yet another skill you can appreciate more by focussing in on it - practicing it specifically by making it central to the movement you are making. Your eyes, ears and feet all get involved in balancing activities.

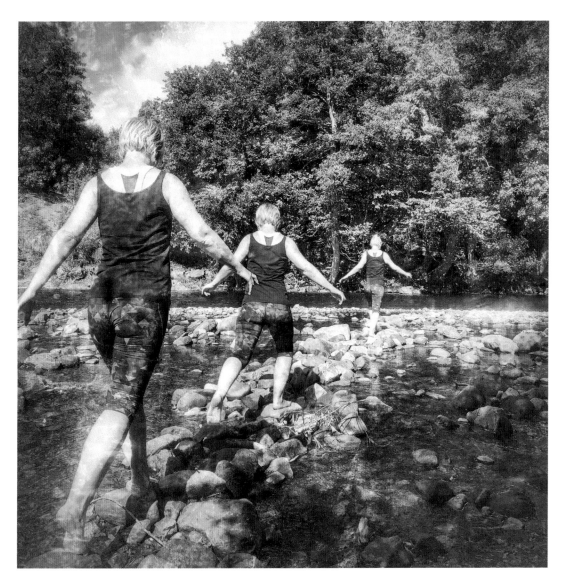

Your arms may even rise up and lend a hand if they think you need it.

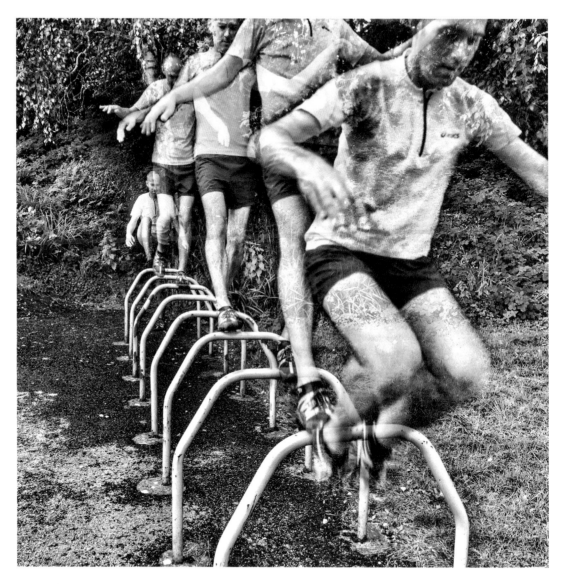

The more you practice the more you notice your mind observing and enjoying the experience, rather than trying to control it. You feel more centred and relaxed. Well balanced.

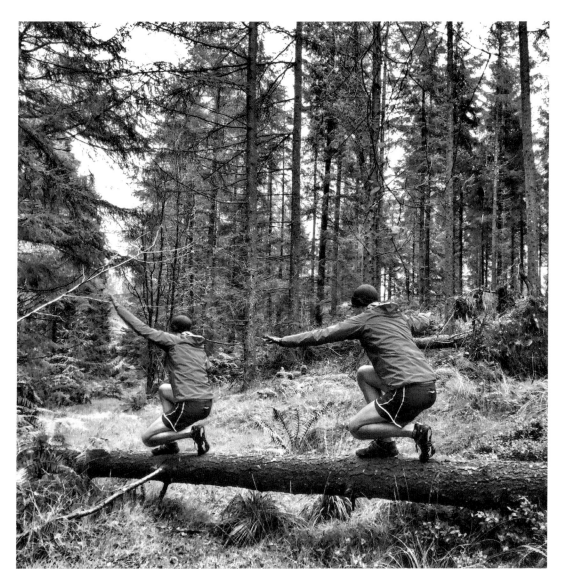

This improved connection between body and mind - this sense of balance - helps you develop confidence to tackle challenges where you may not be completely in control. Both in movement and in life.

leap

"Once you have tasted flight,
you will forever walk the earth with
your eyes turned skyward, for there
you have been, and there you will
always long to return."

— Leonardo da Vinci

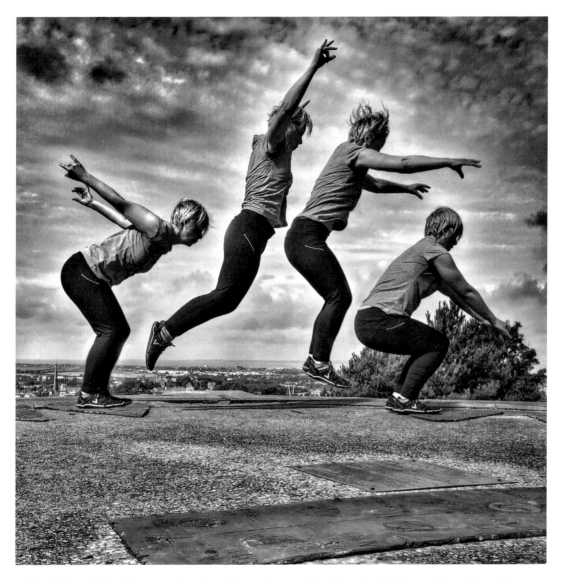

Your biggest challenge so far. Jumping asks your body and mind a number of questions. Not least; are you comfortable leaving the ground completely, and are you confident in your ability to come back down?

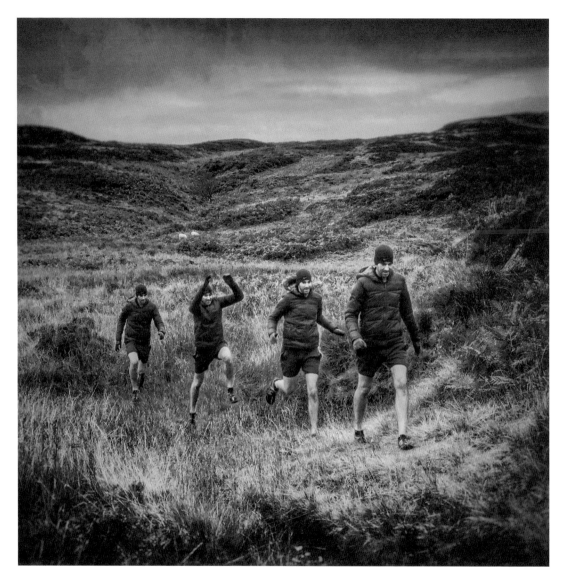

Initially it's more about rediscovering your natural bounce than an ability to generate explosive power. As you find yourself walking with more spring in your step, your next step could just as easily be a small jump.

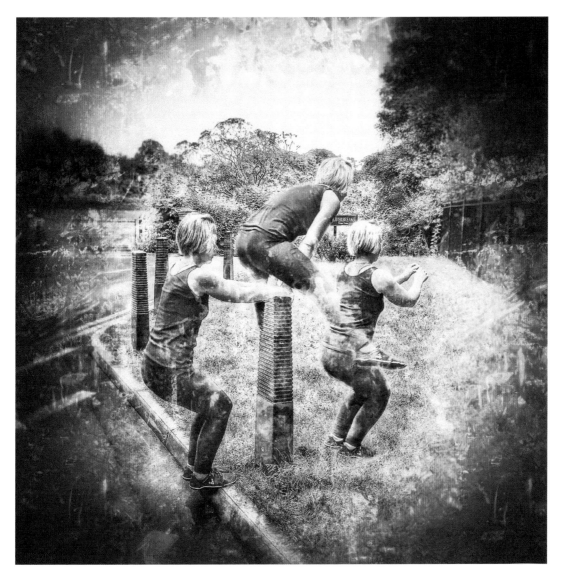

Coil, uncoil, re-coil. Take off is important and often requires a little courage, but the real art of jumping is in landing well - reloading the spring safely - ready to continue immediately on your way.

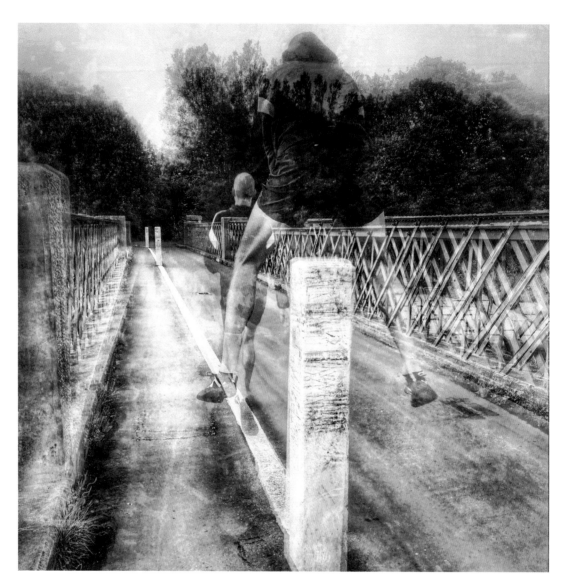

Eventually you may like to try adding a little spring to those obstacles you met previously. Use your body and whatever the world provides to help you launch.

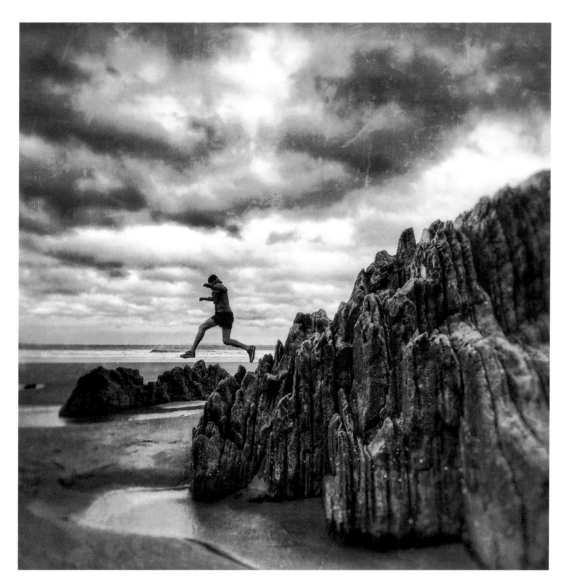

You never know, one day you might be able to fly.

run

"Dwell on the beauty of life.
Watch the stars, and see
yourself running with them."

— Marcus Aurelius

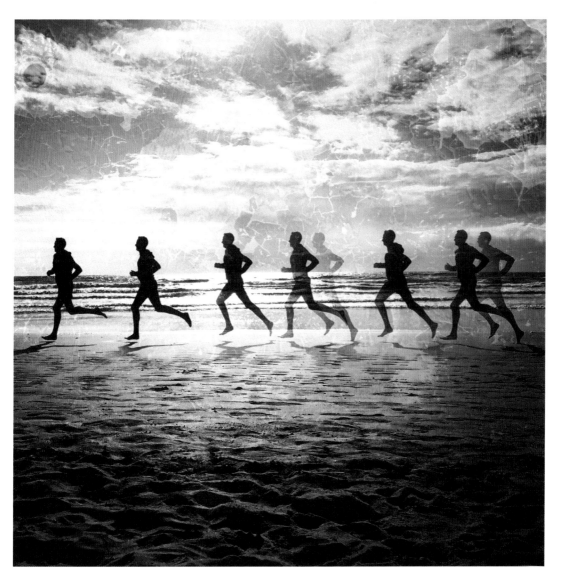

You're having fun now. Your movement range is increasing, you're more balanced, more springy and your confidence is building. All of a sudden you're running.

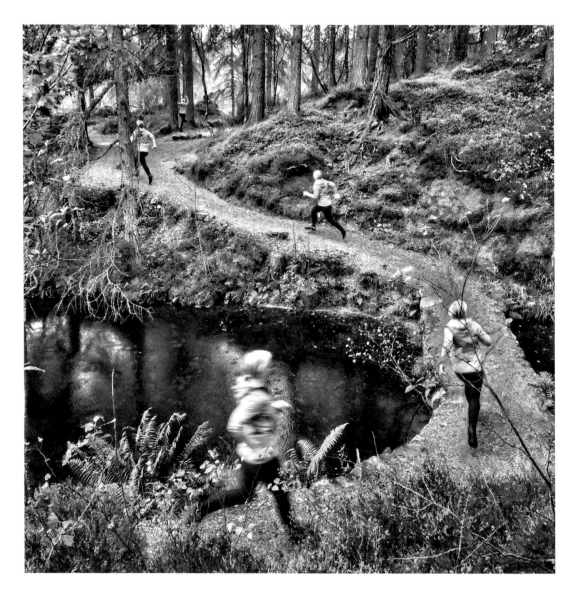

Adding a little running here or there into your movement adventures can get the blood flowing and be truly liberating. It really need not be anything more than that. Let your body and breathing be your guide and see how you go.

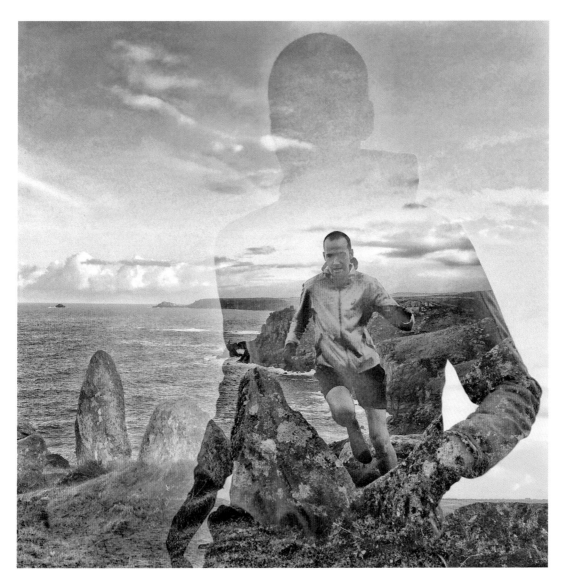

No matter your pace, always aim for a pitter-patter rather than a plod. Feel your senses come alive as you move a little more skilfully across uneven terrain.

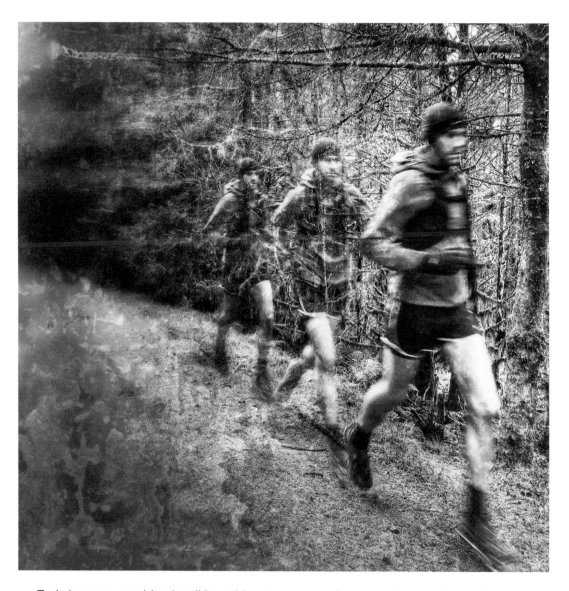

Early humans combined walking with very easy running to explore and hunt. They had incredible range because of how efficiently they moved, skimming smoothly along the ground.

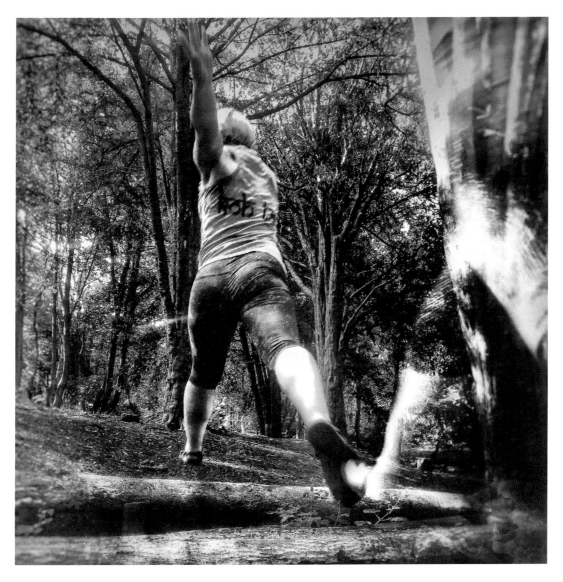

They also needed a quick burst of speed to get away from immediate danger. Perhaps
only far enough to be able to climb to safety.
Mix it up - bound along like Bambi, race to the next tree - keep running fun.

handle

"Before enlightenment;
chop wood, carry water.
After enlightenment;
chop wood, carry water."

— Buddha

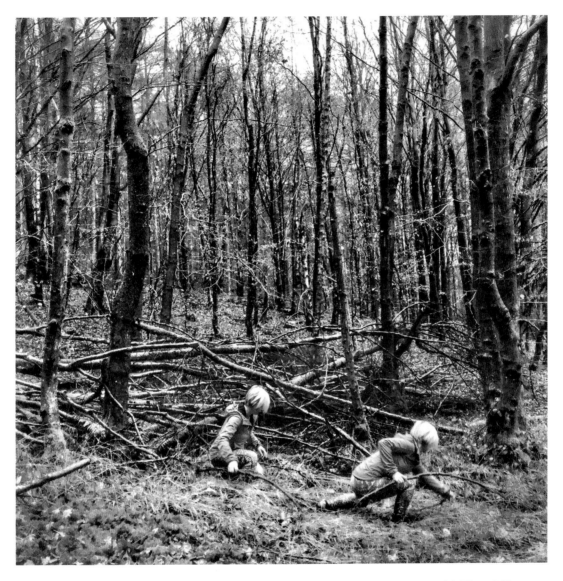

Collecting and carrying objects by hand is a dying art in the modern world. The ability to lower your body to the ground and raise it back up again is one of the strongest indicators of overall health there is.

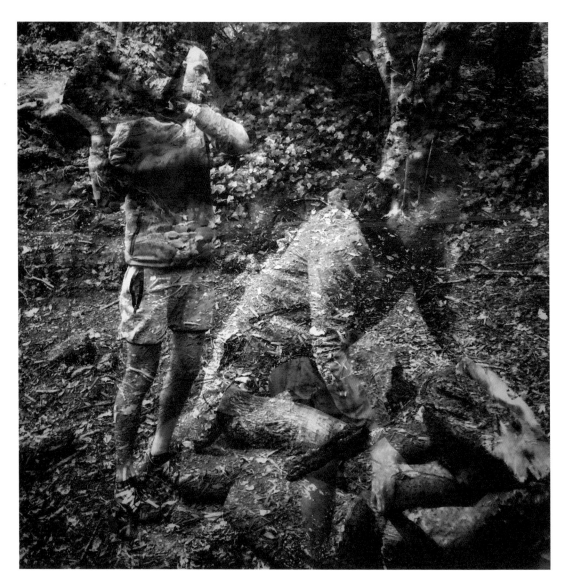

Your ability to lift and carry large, heavy or awkward objects from here to there isn't about making yourself look good in a mirror. It's much better suited to providing help and performing useful tasks in your community.

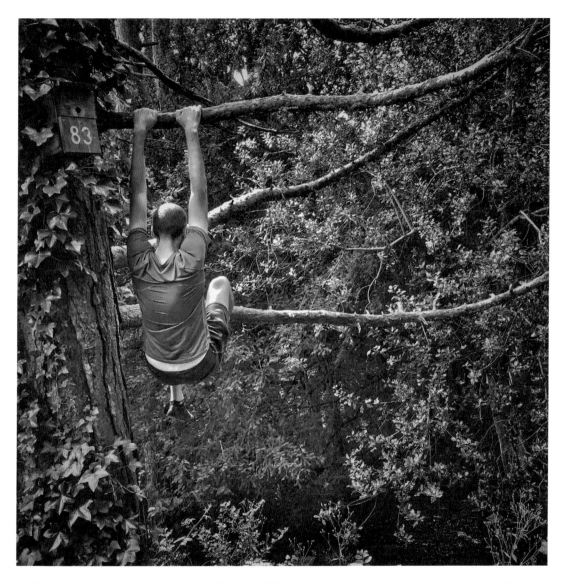

Sometimes that large, heavy, awkward object you need to move is you! Are you able to pull yourself up onto things? To move along purposefully on all fours? Can you be comfortable just hanging around?

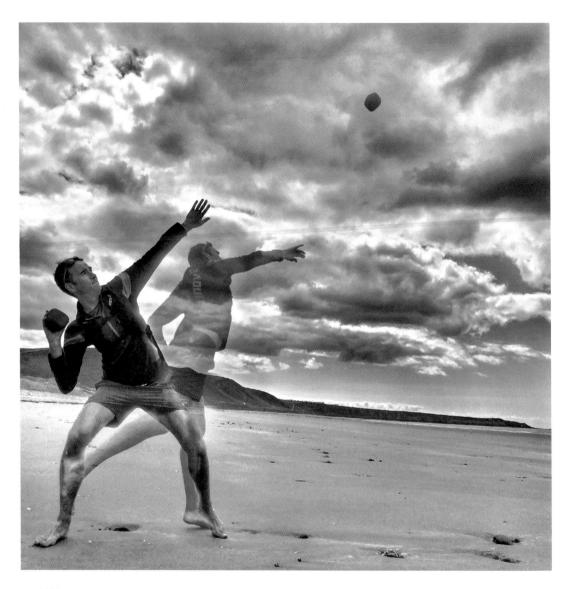

Lifting, pushing, pulling and throwing are all whole body activities. Get a sense of how the rest of your body gets involved with these movements. You'll often find the ground wants to help out as well.

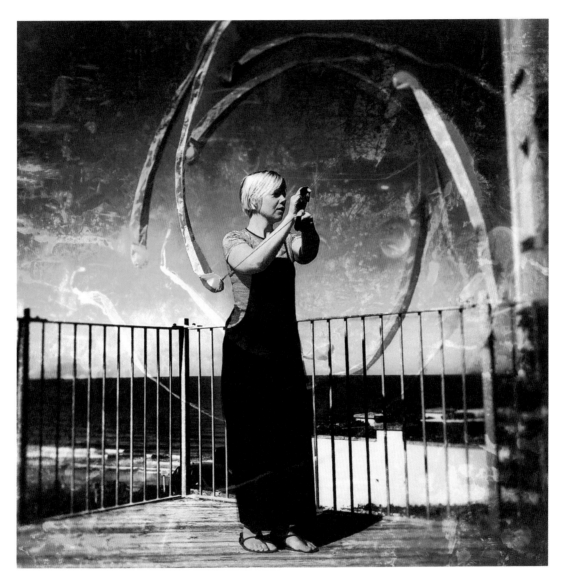

It's not always about moving big, heavy objects and performing useful tasks.
Sometimes it's about beauty, rhythm and flow.

improvise

"Be an opportunist: keep your
eyes open for gaps in time & places
where you can move your body.
Seize the moment. Make stuff up."

— Frank Forencich

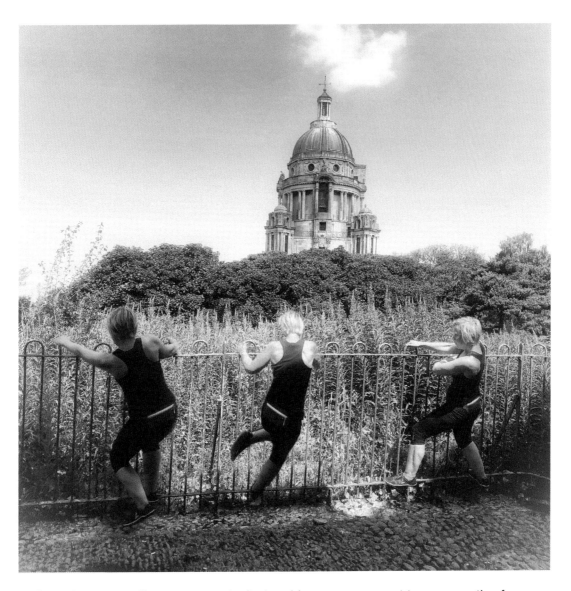

Sometimes you will see an opportunity to add a new movement to your practice for no real rhyme or reason. This also means there is no real rhyme or reason not to do it. Time to get creative!

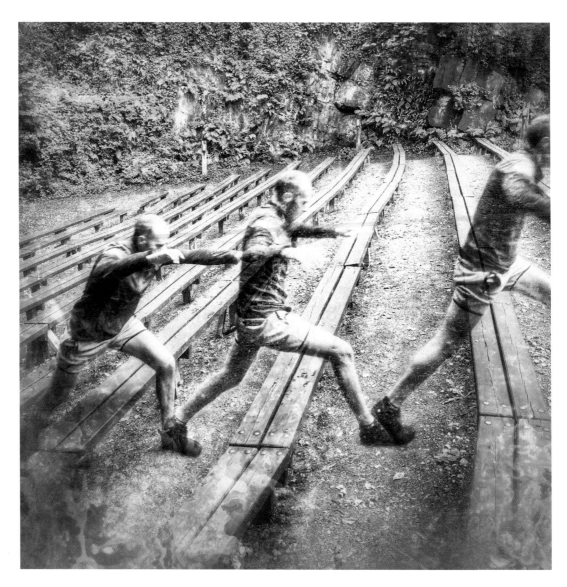

You could stride over something, making the most of those long legs.
Using what nature gave you to help make your way through the world.

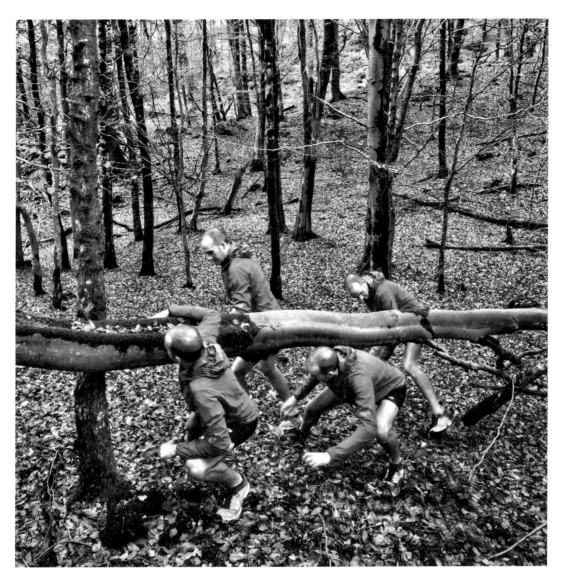

Or perhaps go under, giving those legs a bit of a challenge. You played to your strengths a moment ago, now you're playing on the edge of your comfort zone. This is what adventuring is all about.

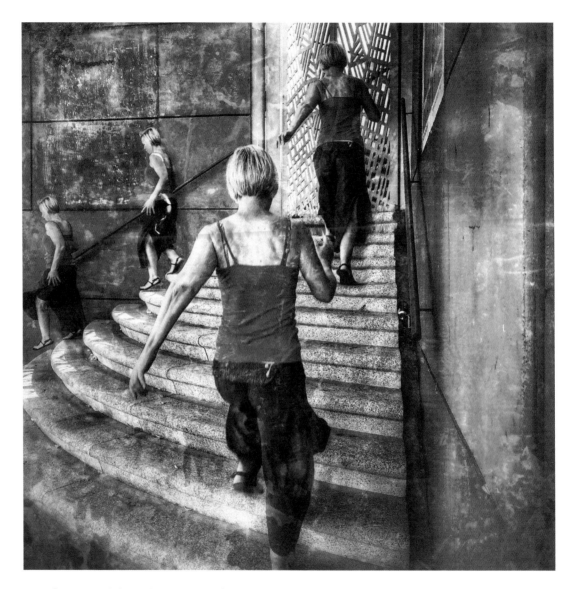

Go up and down just to see what you can see. You can learn a lot about your world when you view things from a different perspective.

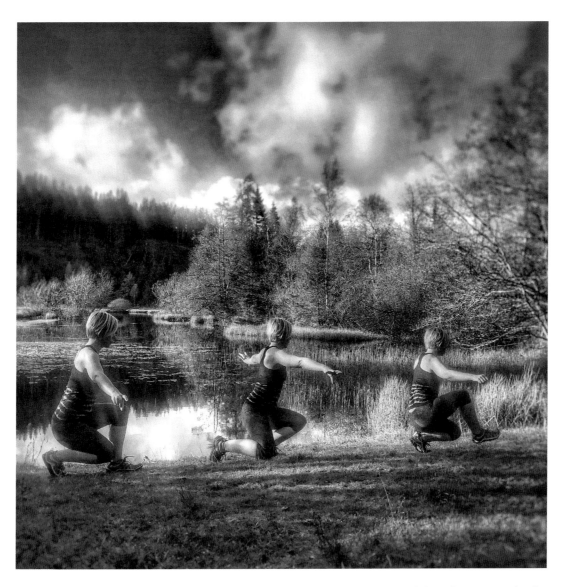

Be ready for inspiration to strike at any time. If you see a tree, a park bench or a patch of grass and think "that would be perfect for…"
Don't hesitate, don't talk yourself out of it, just go and do it.

combine

"The art of life lies in a constant
readjustment to our surroundings."

— Kakuzō Okakura

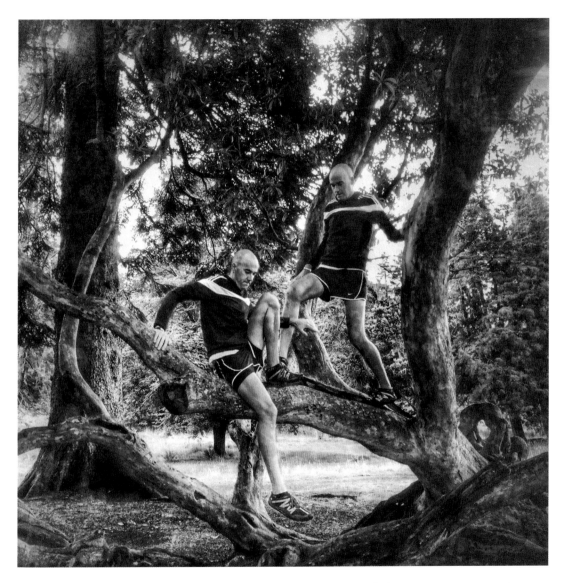

The world provides countless opportunities to combine all these movements you're learning. The more you look, the more you will see.

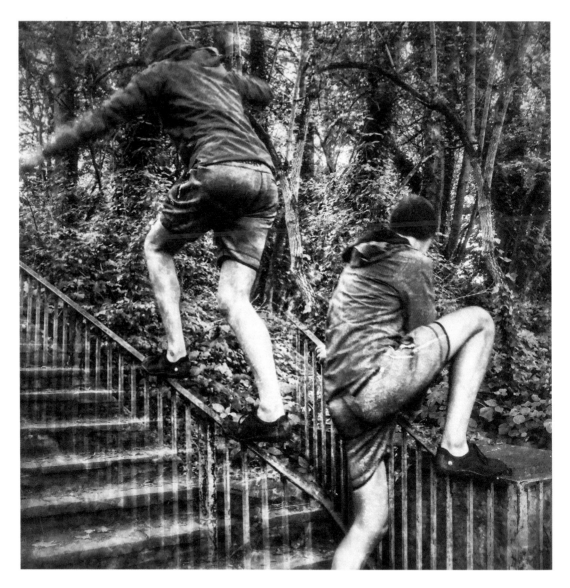

As you learn more about what you are capable of, the only thing holding you back is your imagination.

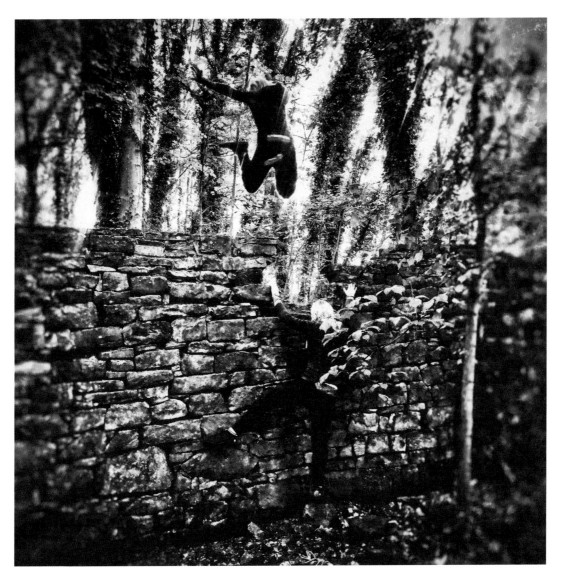

Don't always come down the same way you went up.

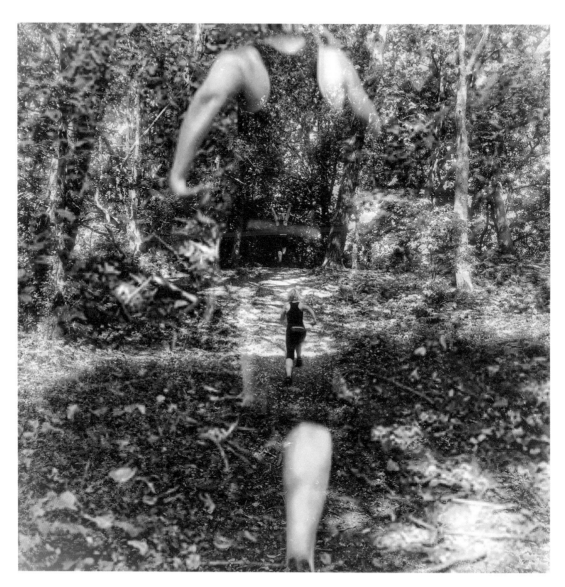

Use your increasing skill, energy and enthusiasm to get higher, faster.

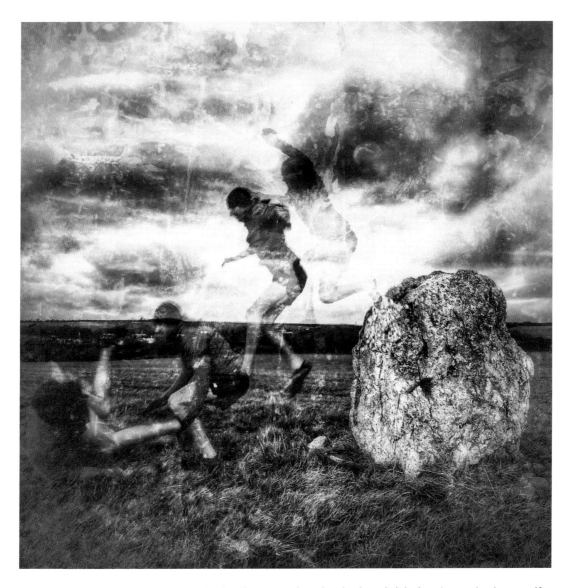

Let your curiosity lead you and take the occasional calculated risk, but learn the lesson if you go to far too soon. Pick yourself up, reassess and go again only when you're ready.

play

"We don't stop playing because we grow old, we grow old because we stop playing."

— George Bernard Shaw

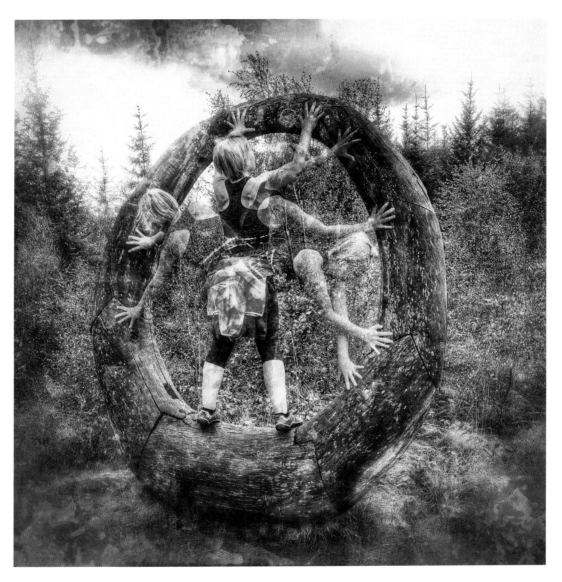

The more you rediscover your movement mojo, the younger you will feel.
Go all the way back to your childhood. Remember what it's like to play.

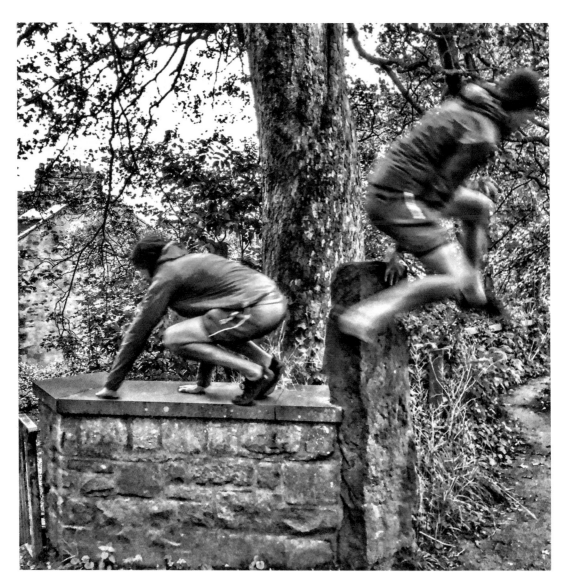

There are no rules to this game. No reps, no feeling the burn, no counting steps. You just have to allow yourself to do it. Your reward will be the smile it puts on your face. Your medals are your cuts, scrapes, grazes and bruises.

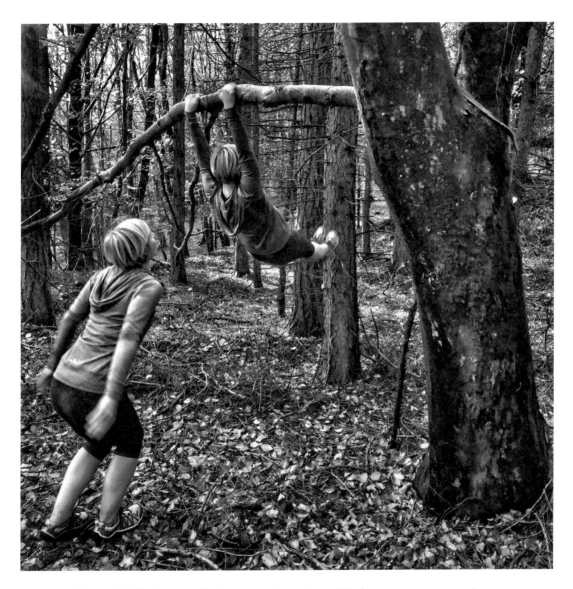

You might find yourself relearning forgotten skills from your younger days.
You may even get a bit dirty. You'll definitely lose track of time.

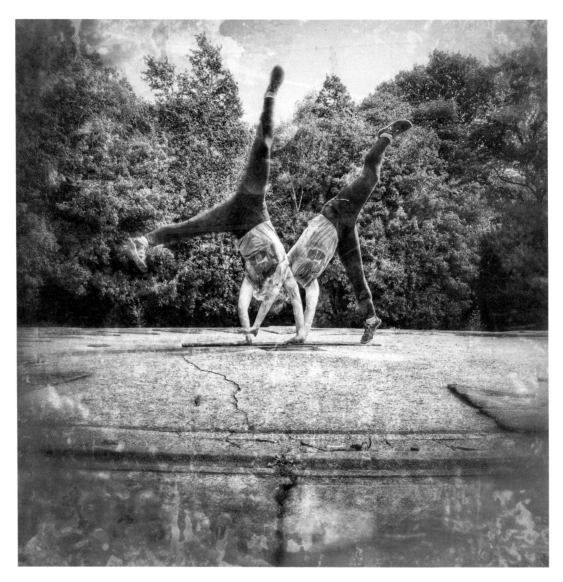

When you let yourself become fully immersed in play, you're having too much fun in your own world to worry about how you might look to anyone else.

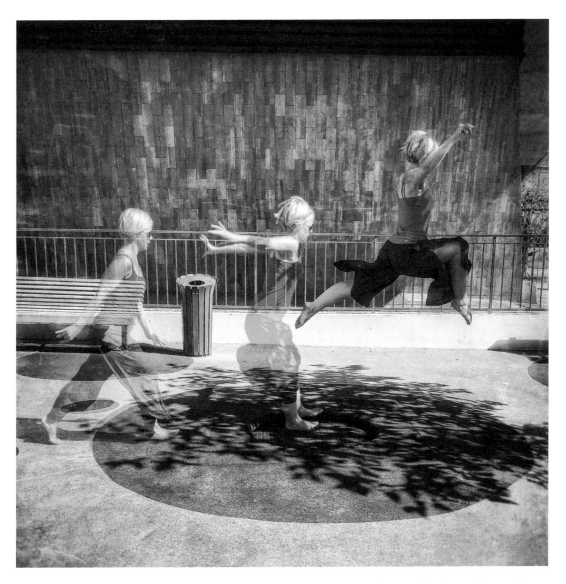

When it's unstructured and there's no outcome attached to it, you simply get better by doing the thing. There is no worry of failure. You cannot fail if you're having fun.

trace

"Life is a series of natural and spontaneous
changes. Don't resist them…
Let things flow naturally forward
in whatever way they like."

— Lao Tzu

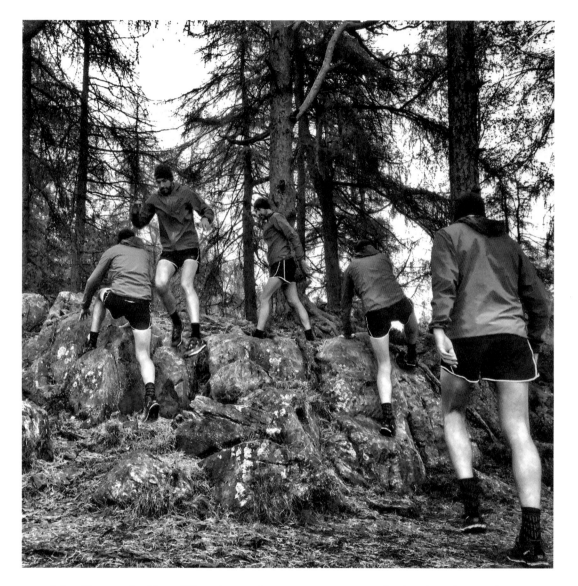

A familiar word with a different meaning - a new movement adventure for you to try.
To trace comes from the French verb "traceur" which means to trace a path.

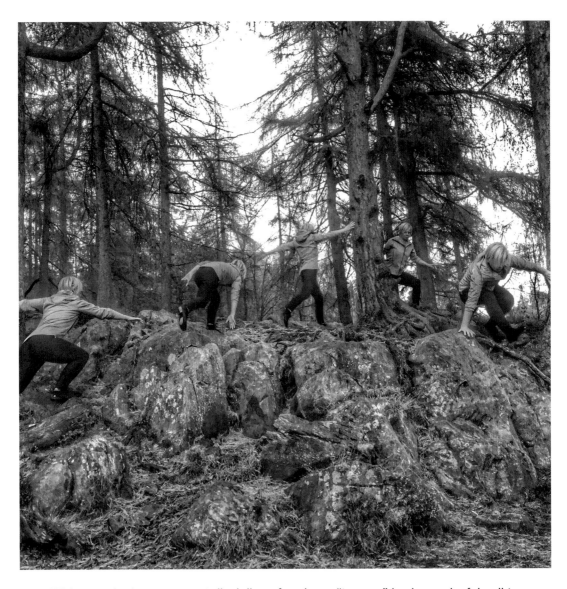

With roots in the movement discipline of parkour, "traceur" is also a playful call to someone to "get a move on!".

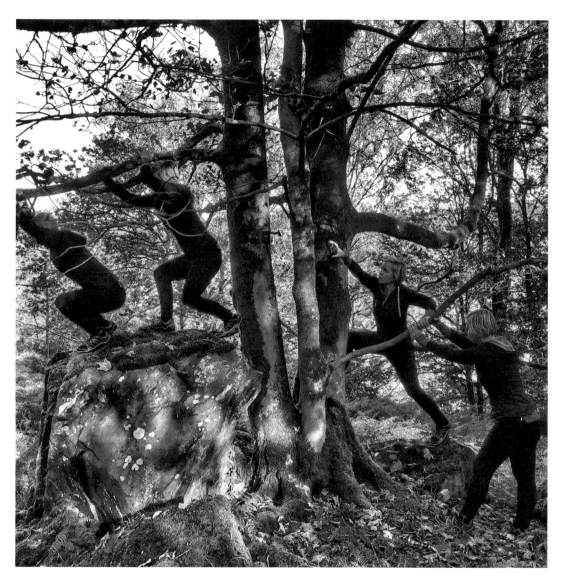

Your ability to make it up as you go - to spontaneously flow from one simple movement to the next - is the true path to movement mastery.

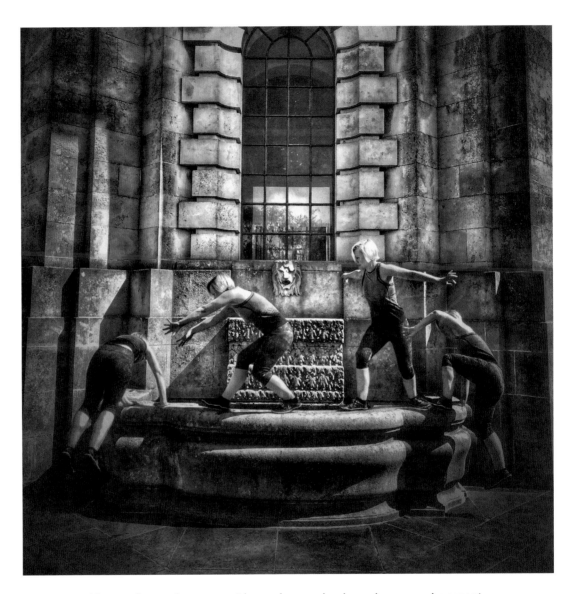

You are becoming more at home in your body and your environment.
Moving efficiently, gracefully and courageously through your world.

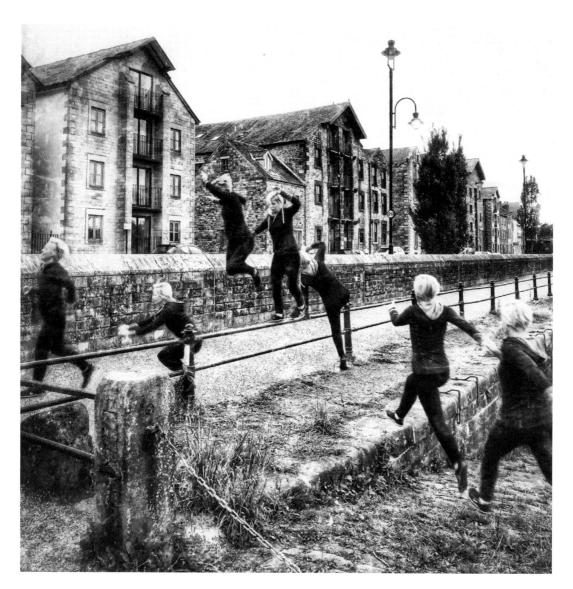

You are a natural mover - truly in your element.

recharge

"Finish each day and be done with it. You have
done what you could. Some blunders and absurdities
no doubt crept in; forget them as soon as you can.
Tomorrow is a new day. You shall begin it serenely and with
too high a spirit to be encumbered with your old nonsense."

— Ralph Waldo Emerson

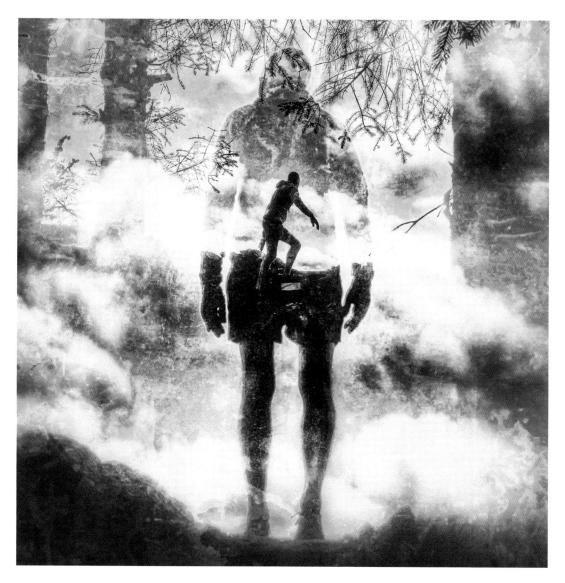

We finish up back where we started, with a moment of stillness and awareness.

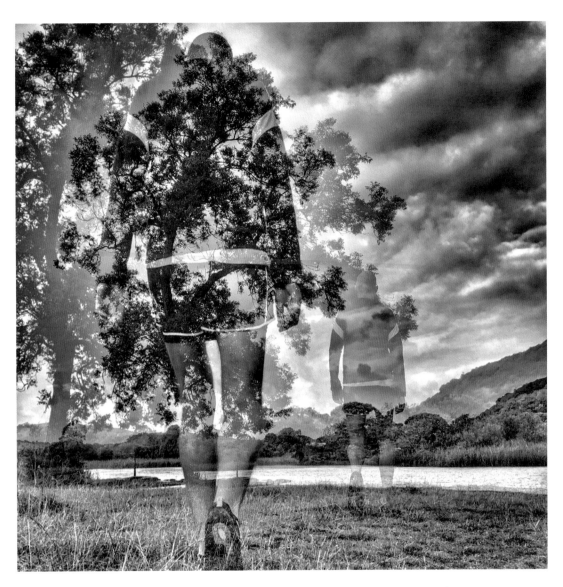

It's time to slow it down for today, ready to rest and re-energise.

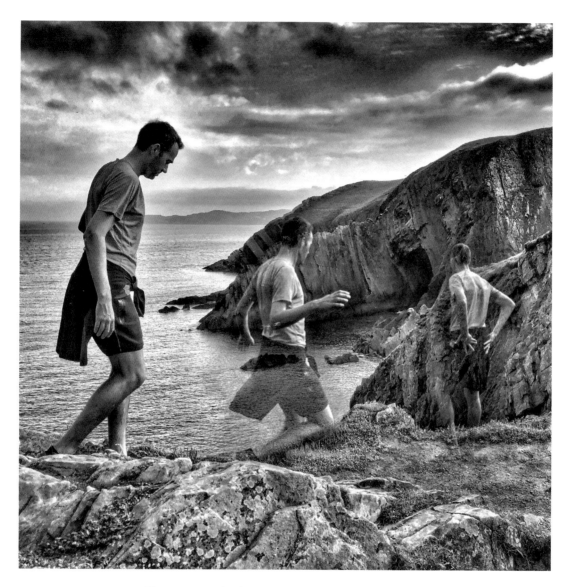

To pause and take a moment to breathe it all in.

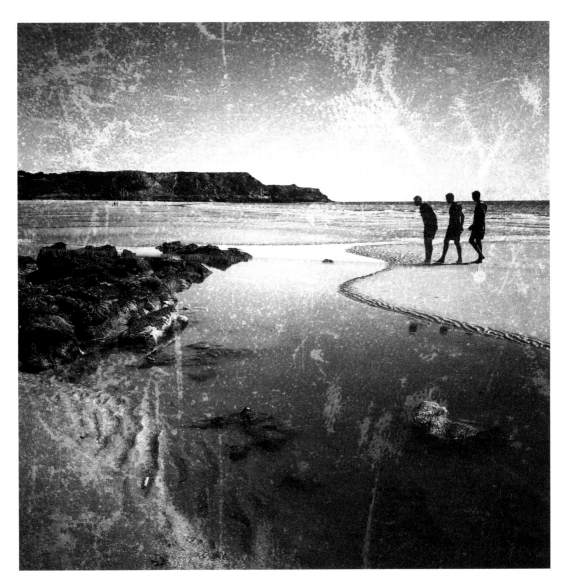

To reflect on how far you've come.

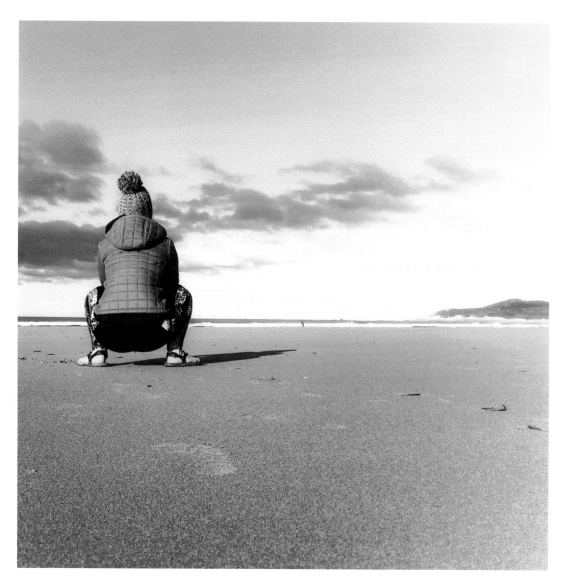

Ready for more adventures tomorrow.

gratitude

"Let us be grateful to the people
who make us happy; they are
the charming gardeners who
make our souls blossom."

— Marcel Proust

Thank you for taking the time to read Move Happy. We hope you enjoyed it.

More importantly that you are inspired to make a start on your own movement adventures. Begin by finding a level that is safe and comfortable for you and take it from there. The beauty of natural movement is that you can practice it whenever, wherever. For a couple of minutes here or there, on a long walk, on your own or in a group. There may already be groups in your area to help you get started. Try these search terms to find out:

Natural Movement; MovNat; Parkour; Outdoor Fitness; Nutritious Movement.

If you do get the bug for moving more like a human and would like to deepen your learning or gain more of a technical understanding of particular movements and skills, here are some books you may wish to try:

A Beautiful Practice & Exuberant Animal by Frank Forencich
Practice of Natural Movement by Erwan Le Corre
Move Your DNA & Whole Body Barefoot by Katy Bowman
Natural Born Heroes & Born To Run by Chris McDougall
Your Body Mandala & The New Rules of Posture by Mary Bond
Breaking The Jump by Julie Angel
Somatics - Thomas Hanna

We'd like to thank the authors of these books for doing what they do and for keeping us moving forward (backward, sideways, diagonally, up, down, over, under and around!) in our own movement practice.

Finally, thank you to Jane, Darren, Marietta and Adharanand for all your help and advice.

—Laura and Dave x x —

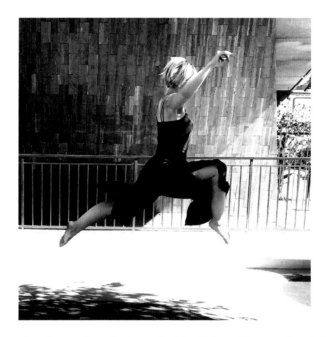

Laura is the photographer & creative designer behind Move Happy. She left behind a career in project management to focus wholeheartedly on her passion for movement & photography. Laura describes herself as a movement generalist. She runs but isn't a runner, walks but isn't a hiker, climbs trees & leaps walls, but isn't a climber or a gymnast - well not anymore!

After seeing a picture of herself climbing up a local monument where she 'felt like a ninja' but looked, in her own words, like a 'big-bottomed crazy-haired middle-aged lunatic', she decided to take matters into her own hands. Laura was convinced she had the tools, technology and skills to make her action shots fit her reality; and from that seed Blurred Edge Images was born.

Laura captures all her action photos using a mobile phone camera, meaning she can literally work 'on the move' & when back at base turns those shots into unique works of movement art - capturing & celebrating the essence of movement in all its forms. If you enjoyed the images in this book, visit blurrededgeimages.com to find out more, including how you can work with Laura on your own projects.

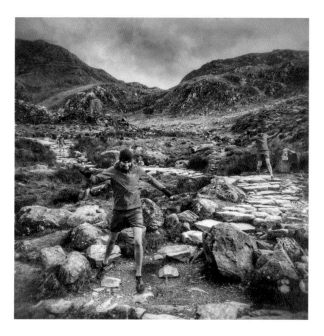

Dave is responsible for the words & narrative thread of Move Happy. He shares Laura's passion for being outside and moving around, but loves to run above all other things. Where Laura describes herself as a movement generalist, Dave attempts to balance movement generalist & running specialist, to ensure he is always healthy and happy in his running.

Dave also left a conventional desk job behind as day-by-day he was feeling more caged - more hemmed in by it all. A simple, playful, more creative life beckoned for both he and Laura. A life lived more on their own terms and one that felt a little more like an adventure than a routine. His biggest take away from the corporate world was a love for mentoring; encouraging others to make the most of themselves and their own lives.

Today, he loves to help people question the conventions they live by which don't seem to work for them - much as he and Laura did. To help them to rethink and redesign their lives in a way that is more true to who they are, especially if that is centred around their running and movement practice. You can find out what Dave is up to - whether it be running, writing, mentoring or his general movement practice at therunthing.com.

Printed in Great Britain
by Amazon